A Comprehensive Guide to Thriving with Chronic Kidney Disease

Empowering Strategies for Individuals and Caregivers, Navigating the Journey of CKD with Knowledge, Compassion, and Resilience

Maggie E. McDonald

Table Of Contents

Introduction

Chronic Kidney Disease (CKD) is a prevalent health disorder defined by the progressive decrease of kidney function. This delicate organ performs a key function in filtering toxins and excess fluids from the circulation, which are eventually expelled through urine. CKD poses a serious hazard since it can lead to the buildup of toxic quantities of fluid, electrolytes, and waste products in the body. In this detailed guide, we will dig into the complexities of CKD, highlighting the crucial need of treating this illness for a healthy and meaningful life.

Chronic Kidney Disease is a chronic disorder that evolves over months or years, sometimes with mild symptoms in its early stages. The kidneys, vital for maintaining internal equilibrium, can be affected by many circumstances, leading to the aggravation of renal disease. The insidious nature of CKD makes it crucial to recognize its intricacies, enabling prompt intervention and management.

CKD can be asymptomatic in its first stages, making it hard for individuals to notice its existence. As the illness proceeds, symptoms such as nausea, vomiting, lack of appetite, and exhaustion may appear. The gradual start of CKD needs a heightened awareness of possible risk factors and regular health checkups to recognize and manage the problem immediately.

Managing CKD is not only about addressing its symptoms; it is about taking a comprehensive strategy to promote a healthy and full life. The kidneys' involvement in regulating fluid balance, electrolyte levels, and waste elimination highlights their significance. Failing to treat CKD can lead to a cascade of consequences, including cardiovascular troubles, anemia, bone health decline, and finally, end-stage renal failure.

The necessity of controlling CKD extends beyond the physical domain to the emotional and mental well-being of individuals. The weight of a chronic ailment can be emotionally exhausting, impacting different facets of life. Therefore, preventive care not only mitigates physical difficulties but also fosters mental resilience and an enhanced quality of life.

Understanding Chronic Kidney Disease (CKD)

Chronic Kidney Disease (CKD) is a complicated and progressing disorder that demands sophisticated knowledge to properly manage its effects on overall health and well-being.

Definition and Explanation of CKD

Chronic Kidney Disease is defined by the steady decrease of kidney function over a protracted time. The kidneys, critical organs responsible for filtering waste materials and excess fluids from the blood, play a crucial part in maintaining the body's internal equilibrium. CKD is distinguished by a deterioration in the kidneys' capacity to execute these vital activities, resulting in a buildup of toxins in the body.

The phases of CKD are determined by the Glomerular Filtration Rate (GFR), which assesses how efficiently the kidneys filter blood. As CKD advances, the GFR drops, suggesting a deterioration in kidney function. The stages range from moderate (Stage 1) to severe (Stage 5), often known as End Stage Renal Disease (ESRD). Understanding these stages is crucial for both individuals and healthcare providers in implementing proper treatment measures.

Causes of CKD

1. Diabetes:

Diabetes is a leading cause of CKD. Prolonged high blood sugar levels can damage the blood capillaries in the kidneys, decreasing their capacity to filter blood adequately. Individuals with diabetes must rigorously regulate their blood sugar levels to decrease the risk of getting CKD.

2. High Blood Pressure:

Hypertension, or high blood pressure, is another significant cause of CKD. The high pressure affects the fragile blood arteries in the kidneys, reducing their capacity to function efficiently. Controlling blood pressure by lifestyle adjustments and drugs is critical in avoiding and controlling CKD.

3. Glomerulonephritis:

Glomerulonephritis, defined by inflammation of the kidney's filtering units (glomeruli), is a substantial factor in CKD. This inflammation can occur from infections, immune system abnormalities, or other underlying illnesses. Early identification and early treatment of glomerulonephritis are crucial to avoid the development of CKD.

4. Other Contributing Factors:

CKD can also occur from situations such as polycystic kidney disease, hereditary kidney problems, persistent urinary tract blockage, and recurrent kidney infections.

Understanding these various characteristics is critical for customizing therapies to target the individual underlying causes of CKD.

How Kidneys Work and the Impact of CKD on Kidney Function

To realize the significance of CKD, it's vital to know the complicated workings of the kidneys. The kidneys filter blood, eliminating waste materials, excess fluids, and electrolytes, which are subsequently expelled as urine. This filtering process is aided by microscopic units within the kidneys called nephrons.

In CKD, the progressive decrease of nephron function affects the kidneys' capacity to maintain internal equilibrium. As the condition advances, the kidneys fail to filter blood adequately, resulting in a buildup of waste products and fluid retention. This impaired filtration adds to the symptoms associated with CKD, such as tiredness, edema, and abnormalities in urine.

The impact of CKD goes beyond the renal system. The kidneys perform a key function in controlling blood pressure, generating red blood cells, and supporting bone health. As CKD develops, these important processes are disrupted, causing consequences such as hypertension, anemia, and bone abnormalities.

Understanding the delicate link between kidney function and overall health is crucial in devising successful methods for controlling CKD. By addressing the core causes and applying focused therapies, individuals can take proactive actions to preserve kidney function and increase their overall quality of life.

In the coming parts, we will investigate the symptoms of CKD, look into risk factors, and address the potential problems connected with this illness. This holistic understanding will equip patients and healthcare practitioners alike to negotiate the challenges of CKD with knowledge and accuracy.

Symptoms and Diagnosis of CKD

Chronic Kidney illness (CKD) is commonly referred to as a "silent disease" due to its slow development, with symptoms becoming obvious only in the late stages. Understanding the indications and diagnostic procedures is crucial for early detection and appropriate care.

Early Signs and Symptoms

In the early stages of CKD, people may suffer few or no identifiable symptoms. This makes it tough to recognize the issue swiftly. However, there are minor indications that may herald the development of renal impairment. These early symptoms include:

1. Increased urine: An upswing in the frequency of urine, particularly throughout the night, may suggest early-stage CKD. The kidneys' diminished capacity to concentrate urine leads to increased urine output.

2. exhaustion: Generalized exhaustion and a sensation of weakness may be early signs of CKD. The kidneys play a critical role in manufacturing a hormone called erythropoietin, which encourages the creation of red blood cells. As kidney function diminishes, there may be a reduction in erythropoietin production, leading to weariness.

3. Fluid Retention: Swelling, particularly in the ankles and around the eyes, can develop owing to the kidneys' decreased capacity to

manage fluid balance. This early sign may be mild but needs attention.

Advanced Symptoms

As CKD advances, symptoms become more obvious and can greatly damage an individual's quality of life. Advanced symptoms include:

1. Nausea, Vomiting, Loss of Appetite: The accumulation of waste materials in the blood, known as uremia, can contribute to gastrointestinal disorders. Individuals may feel nausea, vomiting, and a reduced appetite, contributing to malnutrition.

2. weariness and Weakness: The anemia associated with CKD worsens in the latter

stages, leading to chronic weariness and weakness. Reduced oxygen carrying capability owing to reduced red blood cell formation leads to these symptoms.

3. Urinary Changes: Changes in urine color, frothy pee, or difficulty urinating may appear as CKD advances. Proteinuria, the presence of excess protein in the urine, is a typical sign of renal impairment.

4. Swelling and Fluid Retention: Edema becomes more prominent in advanced CKD, affecting not just the limbs but also the face and belly. Fluid retention relates to raised blood pressure and further affects renal function.

Diagnostic Tests for CKD

Timely and correct diagnosis is crucial for adopting effective therapies to decrease the course of CKD. Diagnostic testing for CKD comprises a range of examinations, including blood tests, urine tests, and imaging scans.

1. Blood Tests:

Serum Creatinine: Elevated levels of creatinine, a waste product created by muscle metabolism, suggest compromised kidney function. A blood test measuring serum creatinine is a typical measure for monitoring kidney health.

Glomerular Filtration Rate (GFR): GFR is a critical metric used to evaluate the effectiveness of the kidneys in filtering blood. A decreased GFR suggests less renal function.

2. Urine Tests:

Urine Albumin to Creatinine Ratio (ACR): ACR analyzes the quantity of albumin, a protein, in the urine. Elevated levels suggest kidney impairment, especially in the early stages.

Urinalysis: Examination of urine for the presence of blood, protein, or other abnormalities assists in the diagnosis of CKD and the identification of underlying causes.

3. Imaging Tests:

Ultrasound: Ultrasound imaging provides a non-invasive technique to examine the kidneys and discover structural abnormalities or blockages.

CT Scan or MRI: These imaging modalities give comprehensive images of the kidneys, assisting in the diagnosis of tumors, cysts, or other irregularities.

These diagnostic techniques, when performed in concert, offer a full assessment of kidney function and assist in defining the stage of CKD. Early identification allows for the commencement of targeted therapies, including lifestyle adjustments and medication, to slow the course of the disease.

In the coming sections, we will investigate the varied causes of CKD, look into the risk factors connected with this illness, and address the potential difficulties that persons with CKD may suffer. This complete understanding will help patients, caregivers, and healthcare professionals negotiate the intricacies of CKD with precision and informed decision-making.

Demographics and Risk Factors of CKD

Chronic Kidney Disease (CKD) is an illness that can impact individuals across many demographics, and identifying the prominent risk factors is critical for both prevention and focused care.

Gender and Age Distribution

1. Gender:

CKD does not demonstrate a clear gender bias and can affect both men and women.

However, some research implies a somewhat greater frequency in males than in women.

2. Age Distribution:

CKD is more frequent in elderly persons, with the risk increasing dramatically with age.

Individuals aged 65 and older are at a higher risk of having CKD.

Common Risk Factors

1. Diabetes:

Diabetes mellitus, both Type 1 and Type 2, stands as the main cause of CKD.

Elevated blood sugar levels over time can damage the blood vessels in the kidneys, limiting their function.

2. High Blood Pressure:

Hypertension is a substantial factor in CKD.

The continuous high pressure in the blood arteries might lead to damage in the sensitive filtering units of the kidneys.

3. Smoking:

Tobacco use, particularly smoking, is a modifiable risk factor for CKD.

Smoking adds to the advancement of renal disease and increases the reduction in kidney function.

4. Family History:

A family history of renal disease might enhance an individual's vulnerability to CKD.

Genetic factors may predispose certain individuals to kidney diseases, stressing the significance of frequent testing for those with a familial risk.

5. Other Contributing Factors:

Obesity: Excess body weight, especially around the waist, is related to an increased risk of CKD.

Cardiovascular Disease: Individuals with heart-related illnesses are at a higher risk of developing CKD, as heart and renal health are tightly interwoven.

Race and Ethnicity: Certain racial and ethnic groups, including African Americans, Hispanics, and Native Americans, have a higher susceptibility to CKD.

Socioeconomic Factors: A lower socioeconomic level might lead to reduced access to healthcare services, thereby delaying the identification and management of CKD.

Understanding these demographics and risk factors is crucial in creating preventative tactics and targeted interventions. For instance, those with diabetes or hypertension should be cautious about controlling these illnesses to decrease the risk of CKD. Similarly, lifestyle adjustments, such as smoking cessation and weight control, have a crucial role in lowering the risk of renal disease.

Furthermore, early identification and aggressive care become critical for persons with a family history of renal disease or those belonging to high risk demographic groups. Regular screenings and health check ups can assist in the early detection of kidney impairment, allowing for appropriate intervention.

Complications and Lifetime Implications of CKD

Chronic Kidney Disease (CKD) is a multidimensional disorder that extends its influence beyond the kidneys, impacting different areas of an individual's health and general quality of life. Understanding the possible problems and lifelong effects is critical for designing comprehensive strategies to manage CKD efficiently.

Potential Complications of CKD

1. Cardiovascular Issues:

CKD considerably enhances the risk of cardiovascular problems. The delicate connection between renal function and cardiovascular health highlights the need to address CKD holistically.

Hypertension usually accompanies CKD and further contributes to the pressure on the cardiovascular system. Individuals with CKD are at an increased risk of heart attacks, strokes, and heart failure.

The presence of CKD enhances the impact of established cardiovascular risk factors, demanding attentive monitoring and treatment.

2. Anemia:

Anemia is a prominent consequence of CKD, mostly related to a reduction in the synthesis of erythropoietin, a hormone that increases red blood cell development.

Diminished kidney function affects the body's capacity to control erythropoiesis, resulting in a lower amount of red blood cells and resultant anemia.

Anemia adds to tiredness, weakness, and a poor overall quality of life for patients with CKD.

3. Bone Health:
CKD affects the balance of minerals in the body, notably calcium and phosphorus, resulting in abnormalities in bone health.

Individuals with CKD are at an increased risk of bone diseases, including osteoporosis and bone fractures.

The reduced renal function impacts the activation of vitamin D, further compromising calcium metabolism and bone health.

4. Reproductive Health:

CKD can have implications for reproductive health, altering fertility and pregnancy outcomes.

Hormonal imbalances arising from CKD may contribute to menstruation abnormalities in women and erectile dysfunction in males.

Pregnancy in patients with CKD requires cautious treatment since the illness might offer dangers for both the mother and the growing baby.

Impact on Overall Quality of Life

1. Physical Well being:

CKD's physical consequences, including weariness, fluid retention, and cardiovascular difficulties, lead to a lower overall quality of life.

Individuals may feel limits in physical activity, reducing their ability to engage in jobs, hobbies, and social relationships.

2. Emotional and Mental Well being:

Coping with a chronic ailment like CKD can have a toll on emotional and mental well being.

The strain of managing complex treatment regimens, potential lifestyle limitations, and the uncertainty of the disease's course all add to stress, worry, and despair.

3. Social Impact:

CKD's influence extends to social dynamics, as individuals may experience difficulty in sustaining regular social activities and relationships.

Treatment techniques such as dialysis or transplantation might demand large time commitments, thereby compromising an individual's capacity to participate fully in social events.

4. Financial Considerations:

The financial ramifications of CKD, including medical bills and future changes in job status, can add stress to the overall quality of life.

Access to healthcare services, drugs, and therapies becomes a vital part of controlling CKD and preserving financial stability.

Understanding the complete impact of CKD on an individual's life allows for a holistic approach to care. Healthcare experts, with persons with CKD and their support networks, may collaborate to address not just the physical issues but also the emotional, mental, and social elements of living with the illness.

Treatment and Management of CKD

Chronic Kidney Disease (CKD) demands a complex strategy to treatment and management, involving lifestyle adjustments, drugs, and, in late stages, treatments such as dialysis or kidney transplantation. A comprehensive strategy attempts to delay the course of CKD, manage related problems, and promote the overall quality of life for persons facing this chronic illness.

Lifestyle Changes

1. Dietary Modifications:

Sodium Restriction: Limiting sodium consumption is vital in regulating fluid balance and lowering blood pressure. Individuals with CKD typically benefit from limiting their salt consumption to minimize fluid retention and hypertension.

Protein Management: Monitoring protein intake is vital since high protein consumption can strain the kidneys. Dieticians typically customize protein limitations based on the individual's stage of CKD.

Phosphorus and Potassium Control: Managing phosphorus and potassium levels is crucial. Foods abundant in these minerals, such as some fruits, dairy products, and nuts, may be restricted to prevent imbalances.

2. Fluid Management:

Maintaining correct fluid balance is crucial for patients with CKD. Fluid restrictions may be suggested, particularly in advanced stages, to prevent problems such as edema and hypertension.

Monitoring daily fluid intake and modifying based on individual needs and the stage of CKD is critical.

3. Exercise:

Regular physical exercise adds to overall health and can positively benefit those with CKD.

Tailored exercise routines, considering the individual's fitness level and any current health concerns, can assist in managing weight, blood pressure, and overall well-being.

Medications

1. Overview of Common Medications:

Hypertension Medications: Controlling blood pressure is crucial in treating CKD development. Medications such as ACE inhibitors and angiotensin II receptor blockers (ARBs) are regularly administered.

Erythropoiesis Stimulating Agents (ESAs): ESAs may be administered to promote red blood cell formation in persons with CKD related anemia.

Phosphate Binders: To treat excessive phosphorus levels, phosphate binders may be administered to limit absorption in the digestive system.

Vitamin D supplementation: Given the decreased activation of vitamin D in CKD, supplementation may be indicated to preserve bone health.

2. Adherence and Potential Side Effects:

Adherence to drug regimens is critical for successful CKD treatment. Healthcare practitioners cooperate with clients to establish a clear knowledge of drugs, doses, and any adverse effects.

Regular monitoring and discussion with healthcare specialists assist in addressing any new issues or side effects swiftly.

Dialysis

Hemodialysis: This method includes utilizing a machine to filter waste and surplus fluids from the blood. Hemodialysis is normally conducted at a healthcare institution, and sessions are planned multiple times a week.

Peritoneal Dialysis: This method of dialysis includes utilizing the peritoneum, a membrane in the belly, to filter waste and fluids. It may be conducted at home, allowing greater freedom to individuals.

Kidney Transplant

Overview: Kidney transplantation is regarded as the most successful long-term therapy for CKD, allowing a near-normal life.

Donor Options: Transplants can come from live or deceased donors. Living donor transplants, frequently from family members or close acquaintances, offer the benefit of improved outcomes and shortened waiting periods.

Immunosuppressive drugs: Following transplantation, people must take immunosuppressive drugs to avoid rejection of the transplanted kidney. Adherence to this treatment regimen is crucial.

A personalized approach to CKD care examines the individual's specific circumstances, including the stage of CKD, underlying causes, and concurrent health issues. Regular contact with healthcare experts, including nephrologists, dieticians, and transplant coordinators, supports a collaborative effort to improve treatment regimens.

Emotional and Mental Health in CKD

Chronic Kidney Disease (CKD) is not only a medical ailment; it deeply affects the emotional and mental well being of persons navigating its challenges. Coping with the emotional components of CKD demands a comprehensive strategy that understands the psychological toll of living with a chronic illness. Additionally, creating and maintaining solid support systems and utilizing accessible resources are crucial components in promoting resilience and increasing overall mental health.

Coping with the Emotional Aspects of CKD

1. Adjustment to Diagnosis:

Receiving a diagnosis of CKD can be emotionally challenging. It may evoke a range of emotions, including astonishment, fear, wrath, and grief.

Acknowledging and addressing these feelings is a vital first step. Healthcare experts, especially nephrologists and mental health specialists, play a critical role in giving information, resolving concerns, and delivering emotional support throughout this adjustment phase.

2. Coping Strategies:

Developing appropriate coping techniques is crucial to managing the emotional elements of CKD.

Mindfulness and Relaxation Techniques: Practices such as mindfulness meditation, deep breathing exercises, and progressive muscular relaxation can help individuals manage stress and anxiety.

Supportive Therapies: Counseling or psychotherapy gives a secure area to examine and manage emotional difficulties. Cognitive behavioral therapy (CBT) is a particularly successful strategy in helping patients negotiate the emotional consequences of chronic disease.

3. Communication and Expression:

Open communication with healthcare providers, family members, and friends is vital.

Expressing worries, concerns, and feelings enables folks to feel heard and understood. This, in turn, promotes a collaborative approach to addressing both the physical and emotional components of CKD.

Support Systems and Resources

1. Family and Friends:

Building a solid support system is crucial. Family and friends may give emotional support, aid with practical parts of everyday living, and be a source of encouragement.

Including loved ones in the journey of CKD provides a sense of connectivity and lessens feelings of loneliness.

2. Peer Support:

Connecting with people who are experiencing or have suffered CKD can be useful.

Peer support groups, whether in person or online, provide a forum for exchanging experiences, ideas, and coping methods. The sense of camaraderie in these gatherings may be empowering.

3. Professional Mental Health Support:

Seeking the support of mental health specialists, such as psychologists or counselors, might be beneficial.

These specialists give specialized support in managing the emotional burden of chronic disease, helping clients build coping techniques and resilience.

4. Patient Advocacy Organizations:

Organizations devoted to CKD advocacy generally provide a multitude of resources, including instructional materials, support services, and community activities.

Accessing information from reliable organizations may empower individuals with knowledge and link them with a bigger community facing similar difficulties.

5. Integration of Wellness Practices:

Incorporating wellness activities into daily life adds to both physical and mental well-being.

Activities such as regular exercise, a balanced diet, and appropriate sleep play a part in sustaining mental health.

Emotional and mental well being are key components of a complete CKD treatment strategy. Recognizing that emotional health is related to physical health underlines the significance of addressing both components concurrently. Regular check-ins with mental health specialists, engagement in support groups, and the cultivation of good coping techniques contribute to a resilient and adaptable approach to living with CKD.

Prevention Strategies for CKD

Preventing and reducing the advancement of Chronic Kidney Disease (CKD) is a vital element of managing overall health. Early identification, lifestyle adjustments, and frequent monitoring play essential roles in lowering the risk of CKD and supporting renal health. Understanding the importance of preventative measures encourages individuals to take proactive efforts to conserve their kidneys and maintain optimal well-being.

Importance of Early Detection

1. Silent Progression:

CKD frequently advances gradually in its early stages, with little or no symptoms.

Early detection through routine screenings, especially for persons with risk factors, allows for prompt intervention and the management.

2. Identification of Underlying Causes:

Early identification helps healthcare practitioners to identify and address underlying causes of CKD.

Conditions such as diabetes and hypertension, significant factors to CKD, can be handled more successfully when recognized early, avoiding or reducing renal damage.

3. Preventive Measures for High Risk Groups:

Individuals with risk factors, including diabetes, hypertension, and a family history of kidney disease, benefit considerably from regular testing.

Targeted preventative interventions can be undertaken based on early identification, minimizing the chance of problems.

Lifestyle Modifications for Prevention

1. Healthy Eating Habits:

Adopting a balanced and kidney friendly diet is crucial to avoiding CKD.

Emphasizing fruits, vegetables, whole grains, and lean proteins while regulating salt, sugar, and processed diets enhances kidney health.

2. Hydration Practices:

Maintaining proper water is critical for kidney function.

Regular water intake helps remove toxins and waste products from the body, lessening the stress on the kidneys.

3. Weight Management:

Maintaining a healthy weight is a preventative approach for CKD, especially for persons with obesity.

Weight control contributes to overall cardiovascular health, lowering the risk of hypertension and diabetes.

4. Regular Exercise:

Incorporating regular physical exercise throughout everyday life helps kidney health.

Exercise contributes to weight management, blood pressure control, and general cardiovascular fitness, significantly improving kidney function.

5. Avoidance of Harmful Substances:
Limiting the usage of tobacco and excessive alcohol is vital for renal health.

Both smoking and excessive alcohol consumption are connected with an increased risk of CKD and can aggravate existing renal problems.

Regular Check Ups and Monitoring

1. Blood Pressure Monitoring:
Regular blood pressure tests are crucial, as hypertension is a primary cause of CKD.

Early detection and control of high blood pressure contribute to kidney health.

2. Blood and Urine Tests:

Routine blood and urine tests give insights into renal function and potential symptoms of CKD.

Monitoring creatinine levels, glomerular filtration rate (GFR), and the presence of protein or blood in the urine are crucial indications.

3. Management of Chronic Conditions:

Individuals with illnesses like diabetes and hypertension should prioritize the management of these disorders to minimize kidney damage.

Medication adherence and lifestyle adjustments are key to controlling chronic diseases and maintaining kidney health.

4. Screening for High Risk Populations:

High risk groups, especially those with a family history of kidney disease, should undergo frequent testing.

Early diagnosis in high risk patients allows for individualized preventative actions and therapies.

In conclusion, preventative measures for CKD concentrate upon early identification, lifestyle adjustments, and continuous monitoring. Empowering individuals with awareness about the importance of preventative actions fosters proactive involvement in sustaining kidney health. Regular contact with healthcare practitioners, adherence to prescribed screenings, and the application of healthy lifestyle choices together contribute to a complete strategy to CKD prevention.

Caregiver's Role in CKD

Chronic Kidney Disease (CKD) not only hurts the persons directly suffering the ailment but also spreads its consequences to their caretakers. The function of a caregiver in treating CKD is varied, involving emotional support, aid with medical treatment, and providing a fundamental foundation for the overall well being of the individual with CKD. Understanding and valuing the caregiver's role is vital for building a supportive and resilient care environment.

Understanding the Caregiver's Role

1. Comprehensive Support:

Caregivers play a vital role in providing complete assistance to patients with CKD.

Understanding the complexity of CKD, including its physical and emotional elements, empowers caregivers to offer individualized help.

2. Advocacy and Communication:

Caregivers typically serve as advocates for patients with CKD, connecting with healthcare providers, organizing appointments, and ensuring the individual's needs are handled.

Effective communication between caregivers and healthcare teams promotes the quality of care and supports informed decision making.

3. Coordination of Care:

Caregivers are crucial in managing numerous areas of care, including prescription management, food adherence, and transportation to medical appointments.

A well coordinated treatment plan is critical for enhancing the individual's overall health and managing the challenges of CKD.

Providing Emotional Support

1. Acknowledging Emotional Impact:

CKD can trigger a range of feelings, including worry, despair, and frustration, for both the sufferer and the caregiver.

Caregivers play a critical role in noticing and validating these feelings, fostering a supportive and understanding atmosphere.

2. Active Listening and Communication:

Being a sympathetic listener is a strong approach for caregivers to provide emotional support.

Encouraging open communication helps persons with CKD to voice their concerns, anxieties, and achievements, building a feeling of connection.

3. Encouraging Coping Strategies:

Caregivers can support persons with CKD in developing and adopting coping strategies.

Encouraging involvement in support groups, engaging in activities that offer joy, and developing mindfulness techniques contribute to emotional well being.

Assisting with Medical Management

1. Medication Adherence:

Caregivers play a critical role in maintaining drug adherence.

Organizing drugs, making reminders, and talking with healthcare professionals about any issues with medications help with good medical management.

2. Dietary Adherence:

Assisting with adherence to dietary restrictions is crucial to controlling CKD.

Caregivers can engage with dieticians to plan and prepare kidney friendly meals, contributing to overall health and well being.

3. Monitoring and Reporting:

Regular monitoring of vital signs, symptoms, and any changes in the individual's condition is part of the caregiver's responsibility.

Prompt reporting of any alarming developments to healthcare practitioners facilitates prompt actions.

4. Assisting with Lifestyle Modifications:

Implementing and supporting lifestyle adjustments, such as frequent exercise and hydration routines, is part of the caregiver's duty.

Collaboration with healthcare teams to integrate these improvements into daily living boosts their efficacy.

5. Preparation for Medical Appointments:

Caregivers may aid in preparing for medical appointments by making a list of questions, collecting pertinent medical documents, and ensuring a clear comprehension of the healthcare provider's recommendations.

In conclusion, the caregiver's involvement in controlling CKD is crucial to the overall well being of the individual. Beyond the practical aspects of medical treatment, caregivers provide emotional support, act as advocates, and contribute to the building of a caring care environment.

Understanding the caregiver's role is vital for enhancing the care offered to patients with CKD and encouraging a holistic approach to their health.

Conclusion

In this thorough reference to Chronic Kidney Disease (CKD), we have studied numerous parts of this ailment, spanning from its description and origins to symptoms, risk factors, complications, and preventative treatments. The importance of early identification, lifestyle adjustments, and regular monitoring as preventative strategies has been underlined. Additionally, we dug into the caregiver's crucial role in giving emotional support and aiding with medical management.

1. Understanding CKD:

CKD entails a progressive decline of kidney function, influencing different aspects of health and necessitating a comprehensive approach to care.

2. Causes and Risk Factors:

Diabetes, high blood pressure, and other diseases contribute to the development and progression of CKD. Identifying and addressing these risk factors are critical preventative strategies.

3. Symptoms and Diagnosis:

CKD symptoms might be mild, highlighting the significance of regular checkups and diagnostic procedures for early diagnosis.

4. Demographics and Risk Factors:

CKD affects many demographic groups, and understanding risk factors assists in personalized preventative interventions.

5. Complications and Lifetime Implications:

CKD can lead to significant issues affecting the cardiovascular system, bones, reproductive health, and general quality of life.

6. Treatment and Management:

Lifestyle adjustments, medicines, dialysis, and kidney transplants represent a varied variety of management methods for CKD.

7. Emotional and Mental Health:

The emotional burden of CKD is severe, and treating mental health is crucial to overall well being.

8. Prevention Strategies:

Early identification, lifestyle adjustments, and regular monitoring are crucial in avoiding and minimizing CKD.

9. Caregiver's Role:

Caregivers play a critical role in giving complete care, and emotional help, and aiding with medical treatment for patients with CKD.

Encouragement for a Healthy and Well-Managed Life with CKD

Living with CKD brings obstacles, but with information, support, and proactive treatment, individuals may enjoy satisfying lives. Encouraging a healthy managed life entails creating a positive mentality, adopting lifestyle alterations, and acknowledging the interdependence of physical and mental health.

1. Positive Mindset:

Cultivating a positive mentality is key to controlling CKD. This entails admitting obstacles while concentrating on chances for growth and adaptability.

2. Lifestyle Modifications:

Embracing kidney friendly eating habits, keeping a healthy weight, remaining physically active, and avoiding hazardous drugs contribute to general well being.

3. Regular Monitoring and Medical Adherence:

Consistent monitoring of kidney function through frequent check ups, adherence to recommended medications, and proactive contact with healthcare professionals are critical components of a well managed life with CKD.

4. Embracing Support Systems:

Recognizing the value of support systems, including caregivers, family, friends, and peer groups, increases resilience and offers a feeling of community.

5. Self Care and Emotional Well Being:

Prioritizing self care, including activities that promote relaxation and stress reduction, is vital. Seeking professional care when needed leads to emotional well being.

6. Proactive Engagement with Healthcare Teams:

Actively interacting with healthcare teams, asking questions, and participating in decision making processes enable individuals to take ownership of their health journey.

7. Ongoing Education:

Continuous learning about CKD, its management, and the latest research ensures individuals remain educated and proactive in their approach.

In conclusion, managing life with CKD is a journey that needs resilience, knowledge, and a collaborative approach with healthcare professionals, caregivers, and support networks. By combining preventative measures, accepting lifestyle adjustments, and prioritizing mental health, persons with CKD may lead not simply lives of management but lives full of energy and purpose. Encouraging a comprehensive and proactive approach helps individuals to live healthy, well-managed lives despite the obstacles provided by CKD. Remember, each step towards a well-managed life is a step towards a better and more rewarding future.

www.ingramcontent.com/pod-product-compliance
Lightning Source LLC
Chambersburg PA
CBHW061008260726
48661CB00005B/2120